10-Day Green Smoothie Cleanse for Weight Loss.

Sip Up, Slim Down!

Lose weight and Gain Your Body Back
Lose up to 15 Pounds in 10 Days!

Tanya Simons

OTHER BOOKS BY TANYA SIMONS

1) Paleo Diet Cookbook for Beginners

If you are interested in Paleo Diet, this book is the ultimate Guide

This book includes 14 Day Meal Plan to lose 10 lbs in 14 days with 100 Delicious Recipes. Paleo Foods to be taken and Foods to avoid and many more about PALEO Diet Also includes FREE BONUS How to lose weight.

http://www.amazon.com/Paleo-Diet-Beginners-cookbook-Challenge-ebook/dp/B01BT87JVO

2) 10 Day Green Smoothie Cleanse For Weight Loss

Achieve Your Weight Loss Goal and Get Your Figure Back

Lose up to 15 Pounds in 10 Days!

https://www.amazon.com/Day-Green-Smoothie-Cleanse-smoothies-ebook/dp/B01E0LMB6A

3) 10 Day Green Smoothie Cleanse. Delicious Paleo Smoothie Recipes for Weight Loss -Paleo Diet Plan Included.

The basic aim of writing this book is to provide all the weight loss seekers some delicious, scrumptious and mouth-watering green smoothie recipes, which help lose 10 pounds in ten days. If you are a person tired of working out long hours at the gym and feel frustrated following any diet plan, then this 10-day cleanse plan is just for you.

https://www.amazon.com/Day-Green-Smoothie-Cleanse-Delicious-ebook/dp/B01E67VO48

4) Coconut Oil Recipes

Best of Coconut Oil Recipes -Most Delicious Coconut Oil Recipes for Weight loss

http://www.amazon.com/Coconut-Oil-Delicious-Amazingly-Beautiful-ebook/dp/B019KI08KO

5) 60 Most Delicious Coconut Oil Recipes and Amazing Health Benefits for a Perfect Weight Loss.

http://www.amazon.com/Coconut-Oil-Delicious-Benefits-Superfood-ebook/dp/B019E3JHL6

ACKNOWLEDGEMENT

I want to thank you and congratulate you for buying the book,

"10 Day Green Smoothie Cleanse".

This book contains 10 Day Diet Plan for you to lose 15 pounds in 10 Days Plus 40 delicious Green Smoothie Recipes to live a healthy life and lose weight.

I hope you will enjoy the delicious recipes and this will help you to achieve your weight loss goal!

Also if you gain any value from this book, please take the time to share your thoughts and post a review on Amazon. It'd be greatly appreciated!

Please visit my book in the Amazon Kindle store "10 Day Green Smoothie Cleanse. by Tanya Simons", Click "Look inside "section and Grab your FREE BONUS".

Else Please visit

https://infinitypublishers.leadpages.co/leadbox/1406b7073f72a2%3A17189 32b4f46dc/5702351037923328/?subdomain=infinitypublishers

Thank you.

Tanya Simons

INTRODUCTION

You've tried a bunch of fad diets, you've tried just "eating healthy," you've forced yourself to eat bland foods that were "good for you," but no joy of eating at all. All you need to do is to hit a "Reset" button and have a fresh start. You do not need another fad diet; all you need to do is rethink your approach to food. You need something that will help you get your health back on the right track, boost your energy, and shed pounds without feeling hungry and deprived.

Our 10-day Green Smoothie for Weight Loss Program will help you leave your chronic dieting behind for good, and embrace a healthy lifestyle that will make you look and feel better.

After a few days of embracing this challenge, you will be 10 pounds lighter! You'll have so much energy that you'll actually want (yes, want!) to exercise. You will start feeling comfortable in your bathing suit and, instead of feeling self-conscious, you will feel sexy!

Sure, green smoothies play an instrumental role in weight loss. The smoothies are made with fresh fruits and veggies and whole foods that will help you undo fast food lunches, unhealthy snacking all day, and ordering takeaway. However, to be successful in your weight loss and health goals, you need a holistic approach to both your diet and lifestyle.

Our 10-day Green Smoothies for Weight Loss Program features over 40 delicious, easy-to-make smoothie recipes for breakfast, lunch, and dinner as well as a meal plan that makes the program easy to follow.

The program will also teach you powerful strategies for embracing a healthier lifestyle that will make you look and feel good.

With this book, you'll gain access to:

The 10-Day Green Smoothie for Weight loss guide plus a 10-day meal plan with delicious, healthy smoothie recipes.

The 10-Day Green Smoothie Program shows you exactly how to use the green smoothies to lose 15 pounds in 10 days, and dramatically turn your health around.

The guide teaches you:

How to holistically change your health around with simple tips for sleeping better, working out, boosting energy, and reducing stress.

Budget-friendly and time saving tips for eating healthy.

Inexpensive workouts that will help you lose weight

TABLE OF CONTENT

CHAPTER 1

10-DAY GREEN SMOOTHIE CLEANSE FOR WEIGHT LOSS.

Sip Up, Slim Down

You will agree with me that most of the food we are eating today is synthesized in a plant instead of being grown as a plant. At no single time did nature ever intend for us to eat from boxes or cans but rather from nature itself (plants) or as close as possible to nature as we can (fresh produce from farmer's markets or your local market, for example).

Eating is a very pleasurable activity that is natural and healthy and aimed at satisfying your hunger. Today, however, diets are the new obsession in the culinary and nutrition worlds (without giving a care to whether they are fads or healthy diets) and this has taken away from the sanctity and holistic ritual of eating and turned it into a guilt inducing and mindless habit – fad diets.

Mindful eating is about creating a beautiful relationship with your food. The conscious coupling of ancient nutritional habits with today's nutritional habits. This will put an end to the complicated and troubled love hate relationship that most of us have with our food.

There are two principles that are at the core of mindful eating:

Attention

Your total attention should be focused on your meal, with every bite, take the time to enjoy each and every ingredient that went into your food, appreciating the nourishment your body is going to get from your food. Paying attention to your food will encourage you to make healthy meals and you are also going to have a better relationship with your food.

Intention

Your primary intention for taking food should always be to take good care of yourself health wise. Forget about over-processed Franken-foods that only make you fat, go for food that is wholesome and nutritious.

Before we go much further, let us look at a very simple analogy. If you have taken computer classes, then you are familiar with this phrase; 'garbage in garbage out'. It basically means that whatever input you feed your computer; you can expect the same output.

In relation to our bodies, if you snack on junk food, you are going to feel and look like junk, but if on the other hand you nourish your body with natural, wholesome foods, you are going to be the perfect picture of health.

The Cold Hard Truth!

Being overweight and obese can result in gestational diabetes – diabetes in pregnancy.

Overweight/ obesity and insulin resistance can be reversed but, if nothing is done about either one of them, it may lead to type 2 diabetes that is irreversible.

When you reduce your body weight just by 10%, you reduce your risk of gallstones.

Increasing your BMI by just 1, catapults your risk of getting type 2 diabetes by up to 20%

Decreasing your BMI by 2 reduces your chances of getting osteoarthritis by 50%

Note: Just search BMI on the internet to learn how to measure your BMI.

About The 10-Day Green Smoothie Weight Loss Program

This plan requires you to eat only smoothies, tea/water, and healthy snacks for ten days.

What to Eat

This plan consists of taking three smoothies, tea/water, and healthy snacks a day for the entire ten days. This will detoxify your body and help you lose weight, with an expected weight loss of about ten to fifteen pounds.

Warning: You should only stay on this detox diet for ten days and not more than fourteen days.

Green smoothies – The Ingredients

All the ingredients should be raw. Only use fresh or frozen fruits, green leafy vegetables, and water in the smoothies during the ten-day detox.

Use the dark green leafy veggies such as spinach, mustard greens, lettuce, kale, dandelion greens, collard greens, beet greens, arugula, carrot top leaves, watercress, turnip greens and spring greens.

For a better taste, discard the stems for the greens.

Alternate greens to avoid the build-up of harmful amounts of alkaloids.

These green smoothies supply good amounts of protein, but if you feel like you need more protein because of a heavy workout, you can add ¼ cup of protein powder to the blender.

Use fruits such as apples, blueberries, bananas, grapes, mixed berries, mangos, strawberries, pineapples, and peaches.

If you have candida or you are diabetic, use low-sugar fruits such as lemons, limes, grapefruits, apples, cranberries, strawberries, cherries, blue berries, and goji berries.

Use either fresh or frozen fruits, but they must be ripe.

For extra dose of nutrients, add superfoods such as acai berries and mace.

Include ground flaxseeds in most of your recipes.

Use stevia as a natural sweetener instead of sugar.

Use organic ingredients as much as you can. However, if finding organic ingredients is hard, wash off waxes and pesticides as much as you can, using vinegar and scrubbing carefully.

Use purified or spring water in all smoothies.

Green smoothies – The Directions

Drink up to 60 ounces of smoothies per day.

Prepare green smoothies enough for the entire day in the morning and pack up to take it with you.

Drink the smoothies as you get hungry or sip 12 to 16 ounces every 4 hours throughout the day.

Try chewing your smoothies as much as you can to avoid bloating and gas.

Chew your smoothies as much as possible, to avoid gas and bloating

You may snack on healthy foods such as crunchy veggies, raw and unsalted nuts and seeds, unsweetened peanut butter, cucumbers, celery and apples throughout the day.

Foods You Should Use During the Challenge

Veggies

All dark leafy green vegetables, asparagus, cauliflower, cabbage, Brussels sprouts, broccoli, carrots, celery, kale, lettuce, spinach, collards, cucumbers, parsley, zucchini

Fruits

All fresh fruits are healthy. However, for weight loss, choose low-sugar fruits such as grapefruits, blueberries, blackberries, cranberries, strawberries, raspberries, passion fruit, limes, lemons.

Milk

Almond milk, coconut milk, hemp milk, goat's milk, oat milk

Nuts and seeds (Raw and unsalted)

Nuts: almonds, cedar nuts, cashews, macadamia, hazelnuts, pecans, peanuts, Brazil nuts, pistachios, walnuts

Seeds: sunflower seeds, pumpkin seeds, hemp seeds, flaxseeds, chia seeds, sesame seeds.

Oils

Extra virgin olive oil, coconut oil, avocado oil, fish oil, flaxseed oil, sesame oil

Sweeteners

Stevia or raw honey

Snacks

Fresh fruits & veggies, lightly salted popcorn, nuts and seeds, organic unsweetened chocolate, almond butter, cashew butter/ peanut butter

Beverages

Spring or distilled water, coconut water, fresh-squeezed juices, green tea, black tea, mint tea/ other herbal teas

Superfood Additions for Smoothies

Aloe Vera, acai berries, avocado, chia seeds, cayenne pepper, goji berries, ginger, flaxseed oil, coconut oil, raw chocolate, fresh wheatgrass juice, sprouts, maca root, or pomegranate juice

Foods to Avoid on the Program

During the challenge, avoid starchy veggies such as beets, carrots, sweet potatoes, and all non-leafy greens.

Processed and refined foods

Refined sugar

Refined carbs such as pastas, breads, donuts, etc.

Animal foods such as meats

Dairy such as milk, cheese, cream, butter, etc.

Dehydrating beverages such as coffee, liquor, beer, sodas, diet sodas, etc.

Fried foods

Your Daily Routine

Start your day off by taking 2 to 3 glasses of water to replenish what you lost overnight.

Follow with one cup of detox tea (herbal teas such as matcha green tea, ginger tea, peppermint tea, chamomile tea, ginseng tea, dandelion tea, etc.), to cleanse your kidneys and liver. You may want to add stevia to your tea to enhance the taste.

Make sure you drink at least 8 glasses of water as well as detox tea per day during the ten-day detox period.

For the first two to four days, you'll fee irritable and hungry. Snack on the healthy foods mentioned earlier to help your body adjust to less and healthy foods. Snacking will help you overcome hunger, but overdoing it will hinder you from losing weight.

You may experience typical detoxification symptoms such as irritability, skin rashes, muscle aches, fatigue, cravings, nausea, pains and headaches.

In case of very strong detox symptoms, follow these guidelines:

Adjust the ratio of vegetables to fruits –begin with 70% fruit to 30% veggies and work your way up to less fruit and more greens over time.

Keep hydrated –drink a lot of water to help ease the detox process.

Ease slowly into the full detox –on the first day, drink a glass of green smoothie for breakfast and have light, healthy meals for both lunch and dinner (salads). By healthy, I mean, avoid dairy, meats, and sugar. On the second day, take green smoothies for both breakfast and lunch and a light healthy meal for dinner. By the third day, you'll be fine to resume with the smoothies all day.

Summary of Your Daily Schedule:

- 6:30 AM: Drink 2 to 3 glasses of water

- 6:45 AM: Morning Walk

- 7 AM: Breakfast Smoothie

- 10 AM: Healthy Morning Snack + 2 to 3 glasses of water

- 1:30 PM: Lunch Smoothie

- 3 PM: Healthy PM Snack + 2 to 3 glasses of water

- 4:30 PM: Evening Walk

- 6:30 PM: Dinner Smoothie (drink your dinner smoothie at least 2 hours before bedtime)

- 8:30 PM: Healthy Bedtime Snack + 2 to 3 glasses of water

Breaking the Program

To stay on the right track, avoid going back to eating whole foods right after the ten-day cleanse. Start with salads for at least three days after completing the challenge before introducing whole foods. Continue drinking the green smoothies and check which foods are fine with you. Within the first two days after the challenge, drink a glass of smoothie for breakfast and eat sautéed veggies or salads for lunch and dinner. The objective is to eat light and healthy meals. On the third day after the detox, have a glass of smoothie for breakfast and light meals such as salads and lean healthy meats such as chicken or fish for lunch and dinner. Introduce whole foods on the fourth day but keep them light and healthy.

To maintain long tern weight loss, make it a habit to start your day with a glass of green smoothie for breakfast.

How to Continue Losing Weight after the 10-Day Challenge

Continue losing at least two pounds a week by drinking two green smoothies per day and eating at least one high-protein meal.

Health Benefits of the 10-Day Green Smoothie Weight Loss Program

Besides weight loss, our 10-day green smoothie weight loss program reduces the risks for: constipation, bloating, allergies, brain fog, headaches, food cravings, indigestion, yeast infections, sensitivities, chronic pain, and insomnia.

As usual, this program is not designed to place any professional medical treatment for any condition. Consult your physician before embarking on the program.

The 10-Day Green Smoothie Weight Loss Meal Plan

Your Daily Meal Guide

Keep an eye on the amount of calories you consume for each meal to achieve your weight loss target.

Women (daily allowance 1400kcal)

- Breakfast: 280kcal

- Lunch: 420kcal

- Dinner: 420kcal

- Snacks: 280kcal

Men (daily allowance 1,900kcal)

- Breakfast: 380kcal

- Lunch: 570kcal

- Dinner: 570kcal

- Snacks: 380kcal

If drink more for your breakfast, lunch and dinner smoothie, drop a snack later in the day to stay on track.

The Shopping List for the 10-Day
Green Smoothie Program

During the ten days' detox, you'll shop twice: shopping for the first five days and the last five days of the detox period as follows: And each recipe will be made once in the morning and drunk throughout the day (serving is for one person). You may also want to make the smoothies three times a day, as long as you use one third of each ingredient called for in each recipe.

The Green Smoothie Shopping List: One Person- (1ˢᵗ Week)

Fruits Greens Extras (Optional)

12 ounces frozen mango chunks 40 ounces' baby spinach Optional: plant-based non-dairy protein powder

12 ounces' blueberries 20 ounces of kale 1 package of ground flaxseed (12 or 16 ounces)

30 ounces frozen peaches 8 ounces' mix greens 1 jar organic coconut water (12 ounces)

4 large bananas Celery/cucumber/carrot sticks 7 packets stevia

4 large apples 1 bag of cherry tomatoes 1 jar of extra virgin olive oil

6 apricots 8 ounces' edamame 1 jar raw almonds

8 green grapes 8 ounces' asparagus 25 ounces' non-fat Greek yogurt

1 large pear 16 ounces' collard greens 1 jar natural peanut butter

25 ounces' mango chunks 1 packet cayenne pepper

4 peaches 1 packet sea salt

20 ounces mixed berries 1 packet ground black pepper

30 ounces' pineapple chunks

2 limes (to be juiced)

1 grapefruit

The Green Smoothie Shopping List: One Person – (Last Five Days)

Fruits Greens Extras (Optional)

8 ounces' mango chunks 40 ounces' baby spinach 8 ounces Brazil nuts

30 ounces' blueberries 1 (10 ounces) bunch of kale 1 package of ground flaxseed (12 ounces)

10 ounces frozen peaches 8 ounces' mix greens 1 jar organic coconut water (12 ounces)

2 bananas 8 ounces' baby carrots 6 packets stevia

2 avocados 5 ounces' celery 1 packet Chia seeds

8 ounces frozen strawberries Cherry tomatoes 1 packet Cinnamon

1 cantaloupe 1 packet Matcha green tea

5 ounces dried cranberries 1 jar natural peanut butter

8 ounces' raspberries 1 jar raw honey

10 ounces mixed berries 1 jar natural almond butter

30 ounces' pineapple chunks Optional: plant-based non-dairy protein powder

3 olives 20 ounces' non-fat Greek yogurt

16 ounces mixed berries

3 large apples

1 large avocado (for guacamole)

The 10-day Green Smoothie Meal Plan

Make the recipes in the morning and have it throughout the day.

Day One: Collard Greens Smoothie

Yield: 1 Serving

Ingredients

- 2 cups chopped collard greens
- 1 cup green grapes
- 1 ½ cups frozen mango
- 2 tbsp. fresh lime juice

Directions

Combine together all ingredients in a blender and blend until smooth. Enjoy!

Nutritional Information Per Serving

Calories: 183

Total Fat: 1 g

Total Carbs: 46 g

Dietary Fibre: 5 g

Protein: 4 g

Cholesterol: 0 mg

Sodium: 31 mg

SNACKS

AM SNACK: 6 apricots

PM SNACK: 1 grapefruit

BEDTIME SNACK: 8 raw almonds

Day Two: Kale Spinach Berry Smoothie

Ingredients

- 1 ½ cup baby spinach

- 1 ½ cup chopped kale

- 1 ½ cups frozen blueberries

- 1 banana, peeled and cut into junks

- 1 apple, cored and quartered

- 2 cups water

- 2 packets stevia

Directions

Combine together all the ingredients in a blender and blend until very smooth. Enjoy!

AM SMACK: Hemp hummus +celery/carrot/cucumber sticks

PM SNACK: 1 large apple

BEDTIME SNACK: 1 cup non-fat Greek yogurt + large apple

Day Three: Kale pineapple Smoothie

Ingredients

- 1 cup pineapple chunks

- 1 cup chopped kale

- 2 tbsp. ground flaxseeds

- 2 packets stevia

- 1 ½ cups frozen peaches

- 2 cups water

- 1 cup spring mix greens

- Optional: 1 scoop protein powder

Directions

Combine together all the ingredients in a blender and blend until very smooth. Enjoy!

AM SMACK: handful mixed berries (blueberries, strawberries, and raspberries)

PM SNACK: 10 cherry tomatoes, sliced and sprinkled with sea salt, pepper, and extra virgin olive oil

BEDTIME SNACK: 1 large banana

Day Four: Berry Pineapple

Ingredients

- 1 cup frozen mixed berries

- 1 ½ cups pineapple chunks

- 1 banana, peeled and cut into chunks

- 1 cup spring mix greens

- 1 cup baby spinach

- 1 ½ cups frozen mango chunks

- 3 packets stevia

Directions

Combine together all the ingredients in a blender and blend until very smooth. Enjoy!

AM SNACK: Steamed asparagus

PM SNACK: 1 cup non-fat Greek yogurt + 1 large apple

BEDTIME SNACK: 1 tbsp. natural peanut butter + celery/carrot/cucumber sticks

Day Five: Spinach Pineapple Smoothie

Ingredients

- 1 cup pineapple chunks

- 2 cups fresh packed spinach

- 2 bananas, peeled and cut into chunks

- 2 cups frozen peaches

Directions

Combine together all the ingredients in a blender and blend until very smooth. Enjoy!

AM SMACK: 1 large pear + 1 cup non-fat Greek yogurt

PM SNACK: 1 cup steamed edamame

BEDTIME SNACK: 8 raw almonds

Day Six: Apple Dandelion Green Smoothie

Yield: 1 Serving

Ingredients

- 4 cups dandelion greens

- 1/2 cup frozen cranberries

- 1 banana, peeled

- 1 apple, cored

- 1 pear, cored

- 8 ounces filtered water

Directions

Combine all ingredients in a blender until creamy and smooth. Serve right away!

Nutritional Information Per Serving

Calories: 425

Total Fat: 3 g

Total Carbs: 96 g

Dietary Fibre: 23 g

Protein: 9 g

Cholesterol: 0 mg

Sodium: 31 mg

AM SMACK: 1 large apple + 2 tbsp. ground flaxseeds

PM SNACK: A handful Brazil nuts + 1large apple sprinkled with cinnamon

BEDTIME SNACK: 1 cup cherry tomatoes + 3 olives

Day Seven: Berry Green Smoothie

Ingredients

- 2 cups coconut water

- 1 1/2 cups frozen blueberries

- 1 medium avocado

- 1 cup kale

- 1 cup mix greens

- 1/4 tsp. cinnamon

- 1 tbsp. chia seeds

- 2 packets stevia

Directions

Combine all the ingredients in a blender and blend on high until smooth. Enjoy!

AM SMACK: 1 cup baby carrots + 2 tbsp. hemp hummus

PM SNACK: 1 cup guacamole + cucumber sticks

BEDTIME SNACK: 1 cup raspberries + 1 tbsp. raw honey + ½ cup non-fat Greek yogurt

Day Eight: Green Tea Avocado Mango Smoothie

Ingredients

- 1 cup green tea (matcha is the best)

- 1 cup frozen mango chunks

- 1 medium avocado

- 1 cup baby spinach

- 2 packets stevia

Directions

Combine together all the ingredients in a blender and blend until very smooth. Enjoy!

AM SMACK: ½ cantaloupe

PM SNACK: 2 tbsp. dried cranberries + 2 tbsp. natural peanut butter

BEDTIME SNACK: a handful mixed berries (blueberries, raspberries, strawberries, and blackberries)

Day Nine: Spinach Berry Peach

Ingredients

- 1 cup frozen peaches

- 2 cups baby spinach

- 2 tbsp. ground flaxseeds

- 2 cups blueberries

- 1 cup frozen seedless grapes

- 3 packets stevia

- 2 cups water

- Optional: 1 Scoop protein powder

Directions

Combine together all the ingredients in a blender and blend until very smooth. Enjoy!

AM SMACK: Handful Brazil nuts + 1 large apple sprinkled with cinnamon

PM SNACK: 1 cup guacamole + celery sticks

BEDTIME SNACK: 1 tbsp. natural peanut butter + celery/carrot/cucumber sticks

Day Ten: Kiwi spinach Smoothie

Yield: 1 Serving

Ingredients

- 1 cup baby spinach
- 2 kiwis, peeled and halved
- 1/2 cup apple juice
- 2 tbsp. ground flax seed
- 1/2 banana, peeled
- 10-12 ice cubes

Directions

Combine all the ingredients in a blender and blend until very smooth. Enjoy!

Nutritional Information Per Serving

Calories: 284

Total Fat: 5.6 g

Total Carbs: 55.3 g

Dietary Fibre: 10.7 g

Protein: 5.9 g

Cholesterol: 0 mg

Sodium: 37 mg

AM SMACK: 1 large apple + 2 tbsp. almond butter

PM SNACK: 1 cup Frozen Non-fat Greek yogurt

BEDTIME SNACK: 1 cup frozen raspberries + 1 tbsp. raw honey + ½ cup non-fat Greek yogurt

CHAPTER 2

MORE DETOX GREEN SMOOTHIE RECIPES FOR WEIGHT LOSS

L ooking to slim down? Start by sipping one of these nine nutri-ent-packed smoothies! Loaded with fresh fruits and vegetables, these easy-to-make drinks will help you detox, beautify and energize in just minutes.

Apple Kale Smoothie

Yield: 1 Serving

Ingredients

- 1 tbsp. freshly squeezed lemon juice

- ½ cup freshly extracted apple juice

- 1/2 banana

- 1 chopped stalk celery

- 3/4cup chopped kale, stemmed

- ½ cup ice

Directions

Combine all the ingredients in a blender and blend until very smooth. Serve immediately.

Nutritional Information Per Serving

Calories: 139

Total Fat: 1 g

Total Carbs: 35 g

Dietary Fibre: 3 g

Protein: 3 g

Cholesterol: 0 mg

Sodium: 36 mg

Peachy Berry

Yield: 1 Serving

Ingredients

- 1cup baby spinach

- 1 ½ cups kale

- 2 tbsp. ground flaxseeds

- 2 cups water

- Optional: 1 scoop protein powder

Directions

Combine together all the ingredients in a blender and blend until very smooth. Enjoy!

Nutritional Information Per Serving

Calories: 79

Total Fat: 0.4 g

Total Carbs: 15 g

Dietary Fibre: 4.7 g

Protein: 1.3 g

Cholesterol: 0 mg

Sodium: 29 mg

Banana Nectarine Chard Smoothie

Yield: 1 Serving

Ingredients

- 1 nectarine, pitted
- 1 banana
- 1 handful Swiss chard
- 1 tbsp. chia seeds
- 1 cup water
- 2 ice cubes

Directions

Blend together all the ingredients in a blender until very smooth. Serve right away!

Nutritional Information Per Serving

Calories: 204

Total Fat: 3.4 g

Total Carbs: 46.3 g

Dietary Fibre: 8.6 g

Protein: 4.9 g

Cholesterol: 0 mg

Sodium: 78 mg

Berry Avocado Smoothie

Yield: 1 Serving

Ingredients

- ¼ avocado

- ½ cup of red raspberries

- ½ cup of blackberries

- 1 whole banana

- 1/2 cup water

Directions

Combine all the ingredients in a blender and blend until very smooth. Enjoy!

Nutritional Information Per Serving

Calories: 275

Total Fat: 8.2 g

Total Carbs: 54 g

Dietary Fibre: 11 g

Protein: 6 g

Cholesterol: 0 mg

Sodium: 63 mg

Berry Banana Smoothie

Yields: 3 to 4 Servings

Ingredients

- 1 cup coconut water

- 1 cup spinach

- 1/2 frozen banana

- 1 cup frozen mixed berries

- 1/4 tsp. cayenne pepper

- Optional: ¼ cup protein powder

Directions

Combine all the ingredients in a blender and blend on high until very smooth. Enjoy!

Nutritional Information Per Serving

Calories: 211

Protein: 3.4 g

Total Fat: 5.2 g

Cholesterol: 0 mg

Total Carbs: 29.5 g

Sodium: 41 mg

Dietary Fibre: 4.9 g

Day Ten: Mango Apple Smoothie

Ingredients

- 1 ½ cups mangos

- 1 cored and quartered apple

- 2 cups baby spinach

- 2 tbsp. ground flaxseeds

- 2 cups frozen strawberries

- 1 packet stevia

- 2 cups water

Directions

Combine together all the ingredients in a blender and blend until very smooth. Enjoy!

Avocado Kiwi Smoothie

Yield: 1 Serving

Ingredients

- 1 cup water

- 2 kiwis

- ½ avocado

- 1 banana

- 2 cups fresh baby spinach

Directions

Combine all the ingredients in a blender and blend until very smooth. Enjoy

Nutritional Information Per Serving

Calories: 379

Total Fat: 15.8 g

Total Carbs: 63 g

Dietary Fibre: 8.5 g

Protein: 6.3 g

Cholesterol: 0 mg

Sodium: 42 mg

Apple Avocado Smoothie

Yield: 1 Serving

Ingredients

- 1 tbsp. freshly squeezed lime juice

- 1/2 avocado

- 1 green apple

- 1 cup water

Directions

Combine all ingredients in a blender until creamy and smooth. Serve right away!

Nutritional Information Per Serving

Calories: 233

Total Fat: 15 g

Total Carbs: 28 g

Dietary Fibre: 9.1 g

Protein: 2.4 g

Cholesterol: 0 mg

Sodium: 54 mg

Kiwi Berry Punch

Yields: 2 Servings

Ingredients

- 1 kiwi
- 2 cups spinach, fresh
- 1/2 avocado
- 1 bananas

- 1 cup mixed berries
- 1 cup blueberries
- 2 cups water

Directions

Combine all the ingredients in a blender and blend until very smooth. Enjoy

Nutritional Information Per Serving

Calories: 267

Total Fat: 10.8 g

Total Carbs: 43.5 g

Dietary Fibre: 10.9 g

Protein: 3.9 g

Cholesterol: 0 mg

Sodium: 36 mg

Minty-Mango Smoothie

Yield: 2 Servings

Ingredients:

- 2 ripe mangos, chopped into chunks

- 1/2 cup fresh mint leaves

- 2 cups baby spinach

- 1/4 cup freshly squeezed lime juice

- 1 cup coconut water

- 1 banana

- 1 1/2 cup ice cubes

Directions

Combine all the ingredients in a blender and blend until very smooth. Enjoy

Nutritional Information Per Serving

Calories: 234

Protein: 5 g

Total Fat: 0.9 g

Cholesterol: 0 mg

Total Carbs: 72 g

Sodium: 51 mg

Dietary Fibre: 6.7 g

Mango Banana jalapeno

Yield: 2 Servings

Ingredients

- 2 cups baby spinach

- 2 bananas, chopped into chunks

- ½ tsp. chopped jalapeno pepper

- 1 cup frozen mango chunks

Directions

Combine all the ingredients in a blender and blend until very smooth. Enjoy!

Nutritional Information Per Serving

Calories: 185

Total Fat: 0.8 g

Total Carbs: 46 g

Dietary Fibre: 5.6 g

Protein: 2.7 g

Cholesterol: 0 mg

Sodium: 27 mg

Raspberry Jalapeno Smoothie

Yield: 2 Servings

Ingredients

- 1 cup raspberries
- 1/2 cup beets
- ½ jalapeno, seeded
- 1 apple, chopped
- 1 tbsp. hemp seeds
- ¼ cup freshly squeezed lemon juice
- 1 cup coconut water
- 1 cup ice

Directions

Combine all the ingredients in a blender and blend until very smooth. Enjoy!

Nutritional Information Per Serving

Calories: 156

Protein: 3.2 g

Total Fat: 2.6 g

Cholesterol: 0 mg

Total Carbs: 32.5

Sodium: 56 mg

Dietary Fibre: 7.3 g

Citrus Aloe

Yield: 2 Servings

Ingredients

- ½ tsp. freshly squeezed lime juice
- 1 cup orange juice
- 1/8 cup aloe Vera juice
- ½ cup frozen pineapple
- 1/8 cup chopped parsley
- 1/2 avocado
- ½ cup ice
- Optional: 1 scoop plant-based protein powder

Directions

Combine all the ingredients in a blender and blend until very smooth. Enjoy!

Nutritional Information Per Serving

Calories: 165	Protein: 2 g
Total Fat: 10. 1 g	Cholesterol: 0 mg
Total Carbs: 19.3 g	Sodium: 8 mg
Dietary Fibre: 3.8 g	

Super Green Super Apple Cucumber Smoothie

Yield: 1 Servings

Ingredients

- ¼ cup freshly squeezed lime juice

- 1 apple, cored

- 1 cup baby spinach

- 1 small cucumber

- 1 tbsp. raw honey

- 1 tbsp. minced ginger

- 1 cup water

Directions

Combine everything in a blender and blend until very smooth. Enjoy!

Nutritional Information Per Serving

Calories: 229

Protein: 3.9 g

Total Fat: 1.1 g

Cholesterol: 0 mg

Total Carbs: 59 g

Sodium: 41 mg

Dietary Fibre: 7.3 g

Matcha Pear Green Protein Smoothie Recipe

Yield: 1 Serving

Ingredients

- ½ tsp. matcha green tea powder
- 1 pear, peeled and chopped
- 1 cup baby spinach
- 1 cup coconut water
- Optional: 1 scoop plant-based protein powder

Directions

Combine everything in a blender and blend until very smooth. Enjoy!

Nutritional Information Per Serving

Calories: 122

Total Fat: 0.3 g

Total Carbs: 22.3 g

Dietary Fibre: 5 g

Protein: 1.4 g

Cholesterol: 0 mg

Sodium: 185 mg

Super Cleanser Smoothie

Yield: 2 Servings

Ingredients

- ¼ cup freshly squeezed lemon juice

- ½ cup chopped cucumber

- 1 cup torn romaine leaves

- 1 cup baby spinach

- 1 banana, chopped (preferably frozen)

- 1 small pear, peeled and chopped

- ½ tbsp. chia seeds

- 1 tbsp. fresh parsley

- 1 tbsp. fresh mint

- ½ cup chopped celery

- ¼-inch slice ginger root, peeled

- 1 cup coconut water

- Optional: ½ tsp. turmeric

- Optional: ½ tsp. cinnamon

- Optional: 1/8 tsp. cayenne

Directions

Blend everything together in a blender until very smooth. Enjoy!

Nutritional Information Per Serving

Calories: 135

Total Fat: 0.8 g

Total Carbs: 28.2 g

Dietary Fibre: 5.4 g

Protein: 2.3 g

Cholesterol: 0 mg

Sodium: 124 mg

Mint Cucumber Smoothie

Yield: 1 Serving

Ingredients

- ½ cup fresh mint leaves
- ½ cucumber, chopped
- ¼ cup freshly squeezed lime juice
- 1/3 cup green tea, cold
- 1 cup baby spinach
- 1 green apple
- ⅓ cup coconut water
- ice cubes

Directions

Combine all the ingredients in a blender and blend until very smooth. Enjoy!

Nutritional Information Per Serving

Calories: 74   Protein: 1.9 g

Total Fat: 0.5 g   Cholesterol: 0 mg

Total Carbs: 18 g   Sodium: 21 mg

Dietary Fibre: 4.5 g

Kiwi Banana Fennel Smoothie

Yield: 1 Serving

Ingredients

- ½ banana, cut into chunks

- 1 medium kiwi fruit, chopped

- ½ cup fennel bulb, shredded

Directions

Combine all the ingredients in a blender and blend until very smooth. Enjoy!

Nutritional Information Per Serving

Calories: 122

Total Fat: 0.7 g

Total Carbs: 30 g

Dietary Fibre: 5.6 g

Protein: 2.2 g

Cholesterol: 0 mg

Sodium: 26 mg

Rosemary Orange Smoothie

Yield: 3 Servings

Ingredients

- 1½ cups orange juice
- 1 tsp. orange zest
- ¼ cup dried white mulberries
- 1½ tsp. freshly minced rosemary

- 2 tbsp. mashed avocado
- 3 cups baby spinach
- ¼ cup raw cashews
- 2 cups ice
- 1 tbsp. raw honey, to taste

Directions

Combine all the ingredients in a blender and blend until very smooth. Enjoy!

Nutritional Information Per Serving

Calories: 311

Total Fat: 19 g

Total Carbs: 35 g

Dietary Fibre: 6.9 g

Protein: 5.5 g

Cholesterol: 0 mg

Sodium: 36 mg

Super Detox Smoothie

Yield: 1 Serving

Ingredients

- ½ cup chopped blanched broccoli
- ½ pear, chopped
- 1/2 carrot, peeled and chopped
- 1 cup Purified Water

Directions

Combine all the ingredients in a blender and blend until very smooth. Enjoy!

Nutritional Information Per Serving

Calories: 68

Total Fat: 0.2 g

Total Carbs: 16.6 g

Dietary Fibre: 4.1 g

Protein: 1.8 g

Cholesterol: 0 mg

Sodium: 37 mg

Strawberry Chamomile Smoothies

Yield: 1 Serving

Ingredients

- 1¾ cups chilled brewed chamomile tea

- 2 cups frozen strawberries

- 2 tbsp. freshly squeezed lemon juice

- ½ cup dried white mulberries

- 2 tbsp. chia seeds

Directions

Combine all the ingredients in a blender and blend until very smooth. Enjoy!

Nutritional Information Per Serving

Calories: 232

Total Fat: 5.7 g

Total Carbs: 48.1 g

Dietary Fibre: 13.7 g

Protein: 5.2 g

Cholesterol: 0 mg

Sodium: 6 mg

Fat burner green Smoothie

Yield: 1 Serving

Ingredients

- 1 tbsp. freshly squeezed lime juice

- 1/4 avocado

- 1 pear

- 1 cup baby spinach

- 1/4 cup minced cucumber

- 2 tbsp. chopped green bell pepper

- 1 tsp. freshly grated ginger

- 1 cup coconut water

- Optional: 1 scoop protein powder

Directions

Combine all the ingredients in a blender and blend until very smooth. Enjoy!

Nutritional Information Per Serving

Calories: 133

Total Fat: 5.1 g

Total Carbs: 16 g

Dietary Fibre: 5.1 g

Protein: 1.5 g

Cholesterol: 0 mg

Sodium: 15 mg

Matcha Pear Green Protein Smoothie

Yield: 1 Serving

Ingredients

- ½ tsp. matcha green tea powder

- 1 pear, cored, chopped

- 1 cup baby spinach

- ½ cup coconut water

- Optional: 1 scoop protein powder

Directions

Combine all the ingredients in a blender and blend until very smooth. Enjoy!

Nutritional Information Per Serving

Calories: 105

Total Fat: 0.3 g

Total Carbs: 22.3 g

Dietary Fibre: 5 g

Protein: 1.4 g

Cholesterol: 0 mg

Sodium: 105 mg

Ginger Spinach Smoothie

Yield: 1 Serving

Ingredients

- 1 tbsp. freshly squeezed lemon juice

- 1 ripe pear, seeded and chopped

- 2 cups spinach, washed and dried

- 1 1/2 cups coconut water or purified water

- 1 tbsp. ground flaxseed

- 1 tsp. freshly grated ginger

- Optional, mint leaves to garnish

- Optional: raw honey to taste

Directions

Blend everything together in a blender or food processor until very smooth. Enjoy!

Nutritional Information Per Serving

Calories: 111   Protein: 2.6 g

Total Fat: 0.5 g   Cholesterol: 0 mg

Total Carbs: 25.6 g   Sodium: 49 mg

Dietary Fibre: 1.3 g

Citrus Kale Detox Smoothie

Yield: 1 Serving

Ingredients

- ¼ cup freshly squeezed lime juice
- ¼ cup freshly squeezed lemon juice
- 1 cup chopped kale
- 1 frozen banana, chopped into chunks
- 1 cup water
- 1 tbsp. honey, to sweeten
- Optional: 1/2 tbsp. fresh ginger, grated
- Optional: 1/2 cup frozen blueberries
- Optional: ice cubes

Directions

Blend everything together in a blender or food processor until very smooth. Enjoy!

Nutritional Information Per Serving

Calories: 111   Protein: 2.6 g

Total Fat: 0.5 g   Cholesterol: 0 mg

Total Carbs: 25.6 g   Sodium: 49 mg

Dietary Fibre: 1.3 g

Green and Clean Smoothie

Yield: 1 Serving

Ingredients

- ½ apple
- 1 kiwifruit
- 2 sprigs fresh mint
- 1 celery stalk
- ½ avocado

- 1 cup chopped spinach
- 1/4 cucumber
- 1 cup purified water
- 2 tbsp. freshly squeezed lemon juice

Directions

Blend everything together in a blender or food processor until very smooth. Enjoy!

Nutritional Information Per Serving

Calories: 281

Total Fat: 20.2 g

Total Carbs: 26.2 g

Dietary Fibre: 10.4 g

Protein: 3.9 g

Cholesterol: 0 mg

Sodium: 52 mg

Lemon-Lime Detox Smoothie

Yield: 2 Servings

Ingredients

- ¼ cup freshly squeezed lemon juice

- ¼ cup freshly squeezed lime juice

- 1 cup freshly squeezed orange juice

- 1 cup chopped dandelion greens

- 2 medium bananas, peeled

Directions

Combine together all the ingredients in a blender and blend until very smooth. Enjoy!

Nutritional Information Per Serving

Calories: 181

Total Fat: 1.1 g

Total Carbs: 43 g

Dietary Fibre: 4.4 g

Protein: 3.1 g

Cholesterol: 0 mg

Sodium: 29 mg

Ginger Spice Smoothie

Yield: 1 Serving

Ingredients

- 1 nub ginger root, finely minced

- 1 cup chopped spinach

- 1 tsp. Cinnamon

- 1 cup Purified Water

Directions

Combine together all the ingredients in a blender and blend until very smooth. Enjoy!

Nutritional Information Per Serving

Calories: 23

Total Fat: 0.1 g

Total Carbs: 3.9 g

Dietary Fibre: 2.1 g

Protein: 0.9 g

Cholesterol: 0 mg

Sodium: 24 mg

Detoxifying green Apple & Broccoli Smoothie

Yield: 1 Serving

Ingredients

- 1 apple

- 1 cup broccoli florets

- 1 celery rib

- 1 frozen banana

- ¼ cup freshly squeezed lemon juice

- 1 cup coconut water

- 1 tsp. raw honey, to taste

Directions

Combine together all the ingredients in a blender and blend until very smooth. Enjoy!

Nutritional Information Per Serving

Calories: 162

Protein: 3.6 g

Total Fat: 1.1 g

Cholesterol: 0 mg

Total Carbs: 38.2 g

Sodium: 44 mg

Dietary Fibre: 7 g

Smoothie Power Green

Yield: 2 Servings

Ingredients

- 1 cup chopped romaine lettuce
- 1 cup baby spinach
- 3 to 4 stalks organic celery
- 2 tbsp. freshly squeezed lemon juice

- 1 banana
- 1 pear, cored and chopped
- 1 apple, cored and chopped
- 1 1/2 cups water
- Optional: cilantro or parsley leaves to garnish

Directions

Combine together all the ingredients in a blender and blend until very smooth. Enjoy!

Nutritional Information Per Serving

Calories: 155

Total Fat: 0.7 g

Total Carbs: 39.1 g

Dietary Fibre: 6.9 g

Protein: 2 g

Cholesterol: 0 mg

Sodium: 44 mg

Mango Kale Smoothie

Yield: 1 Serving

Ingredients

- 12 chunks frozen mango
- 2 cups massaged kale
- 1 large kiwi peeled
- 1 banana
- ½ cup coconut water
- A sprinkle of chia or flax seeds

Directions

Combine together all the ingredients in a blender and blend until very smooth. Enjoy!

Nutritional Information Per Serving

Calories: 265

Protein: 7.4 g

Total Fat: 1.2 g

Cholesterol: 0 mg

Total Carbs: 63 g

Sodium: 59 mg

Dietary Fibre: 8.3 g

Avocado Kale Smoothie

Yield: 2 Servings

Ingredients:

- 2 tsp. freshly squeezed lime juice

- 1/2 cup avocado

- 2 cups kale leaves

- 1 banana, frozen

- 1 1/4 cup coconut water

Directions

Combine together all the ingredients in a blender and blend until very smooth. Enjoy!

Nutritional Information Per Serving

Calories: 160

Total Fat: 7.3 g

Total Carbs: 23.6 g

Dietary Fibre: 5 g

Protein: 3.3 g

Cholesterol: 0 mg

Sodium: 32 mg

Green Fig Ginger Smoothie

Yield: 1 Serving

Ingredients

- 6 green figs

- 2 cups mix greens (kale, chard, and baby spinach)

- 1 frozen banana, chopped

- 1/2-inch piece ginger, peeled

- 1/2 cucumber, chopped

- 1/4 – 1/2 cup coconut water

Directions

Combine together all the ingredients in a blender and blend until very smooth. Enjoy!

Nutritional Information Per Serving

Calories: 228

Protein: 10.3 g

Total Fat: 0.6 g

Cholesterol: 0 mg

Total Carbs: 45 g

Sodium: 1204 mg

Dietary Fibre: 11.8 g

Strawberry Pineapple Smoothie

Yields: 1 Serving

Ingredients

- ½ cup strawberries
- ½ cup pineapple
- 2 hearts of romaine
- 1 cup coconut water or purified water

Directions

Combine together all the ingredients in a blender and blend until very smooth. Enjoy!

Nutritional Information Per Serving:

Calories: 134

Total Fat: 3.8 g

Total Carb: 24.3 g

Protein: 4g

Dietary fibre: 5.6 g

Cholesterol: 0 mg

Sodium: 202 mg

Power Green Smoothie

Yields: 2 Servings

Ingredients

- 2 tsp. freshly squeezed lemon juice
- ½ cup chopped fresh spinach
- 1 banana
- 1 cup raspberries
- 1 tbsp. flaxseed
- 1 cup water

Directions

Combine everything in a blender and blend until smooth and creamy. Enjoy!

Nutritional Information Per Serving:

Calories: 157   Dietary fibre: 7 g

Total Fat: 6.3 g   Cholesterol: 0 mg

Total Carb: 23.6 g   Sodium: 13 mg

Protein: 4 g

Apple Spinach Smoothie

Yields: 1 Serving

Ingredients

- 1/2 cup baby spinach

- 1 tsp. freshly grated ginger

- 1 organic apple, peeled, diced

- 1 cup freshly squeezed orange juice

- 5 ice cubes

Directions

Rinse all the ingredients and blend together in a blender until smooth. Enjoy!

Nutritional Information Per Serving:

Calories: 216

Total Fat: 1 g

Total Carbs: 52.8 g

Protein: 2.8 g

Dietary fibre: 5.5 g

Cholesterol: 0 mg

Sodium: 16 mg

Tasty Detox Smoothie

Yields: 2 Cups

Ingredients

- 1 cup chopped pineapple

- 3 tbsp. freshly squeezed lime juice

- 1/2 cup water

- 1/2 green apple, peeled, diced

- 1 cup chopped kale

- 1 cucumber, diced

- 4 celery stalks, chopped

- 2 cups ice cubes

Directions

Combine all the ingredients in a blender and blend on high for about 1 minute or until smooth. Enjoy!

Nutrition Information Per Serving

Calories: 357

Protein: 6 g

Total Fat: 16 g

Cholesterol: 0 mg

Total Carbs: 54 g

Sodium: 238 mg

Dietary Fibre: 13 g

Lemon Blueberry Bliss

Yields: 2 Servings

Ingredients:

- 2 cups frozen blueberries

- 1 cup organic baby spinach

- 1 pear, halved and cored

- 1 cup coconut water

- 2 tbsp. freshly squeezed lemon juice

- 1 tsp. freshly grated lemon zest

Directions:

Add all the ingredients to a blender and blend to your desired consistency. Enjoy!

Nutritional Information Per Serving:

Calories: 156

Total Fat: 1 g

Total Carb: 6 g

Protein: 2 g

Dietary fibre: 8 g

Cholesterol: 0

Sodium: 15 mg

Super Green Smoothie

Yields: 2 Servings

Ingredients

- 1 cup diced pineapple
- ½ cup almond milk
- 1 tbsp. coconut oil
- ½ lime
- ½ green apple
- 1 cup kale leaves
- 1 cucumber
- 4 celery sticks

Directions

Combine everything in a blender and blend until smooth and creamy. Enjoy!

Nutritional Information Per Serving:

Calories: 308

Total Fat: 21.4 g

Total Carbs: 31 g

Protein: 3.9 g

Dietary fibre: 5.6 g

Cholesterol: 0 mg

Sodium: 70 mg

Cranberry Cleanse Smoothie

Yields: 1 Servings

Ingredients

- 1/2 cup freshly squeezed orange juice

- 1 sweet red organic apple, peeled and chopped

- 1/2 cup baby spinach

- 1/2 cup cranberries

- 1/2 cup cold purified water

- 5 ice cubes

Directions

Rinse all the ingredients and add to a blender. Blend on high speed until very smooth. Enjoy!

Nutrition Information Per Serving

Calories: 184   Protein: 1.8 g

Total Fat: 0.6 g   Cholesterol: 0 mg

Total Carbs: 43.6 g   Sodium: 14 mg

Dietary Fibre: 7 g

Cucumber Mint Alkaline Smoothie

Yields: 1 Serving

Ingredients

- 6 mint leaves

- 1 organic apple, peeled, diced

- 1/2 cucumber, sliced

- 1/2 cup purified water

- 5 ice cubes

Directions

Combine all the ingredients in a blender and blend on high until very smooth. Enjoy!

Nutrition Information Per Serving

Calories: 357

Protein: 6 g

Total Fat: 16 g

Cholesterol: 0 mg

Total Carbs: 54 g

Sodium: 238 mg

Dietary Fibre: 13 g

Mango Smoothie Surprise

Yields: 1 Serving

Ingredients

- 1 tbsp. lime juice (freshly squeezed)
- ¼ cup non-fat vanilla yogurt
- ½ cup fresh mango juice
- ¼ cup mashed avocado
- ¼ cup diced mango
- ½ tbsp. honey
- 6 ice cubes

Directions

Combine all the ingredients in a blender and blend on high until smooth. Pour in a tall serving glass and garnish with a strawberry or mango slice, if desired. Enjoy!

Nutritional information Per Serving:

Calories: 298   Protein: 5 g

Total Fat: 9 g   Cholesterol: 0 mg

Total Carbs: 55 g   Sodium: 103 mg

Dietary Fibre: 5 mg

Healthy Green Drink

Yields: 1 Serving

Ingredients

- 1/2 cup diced frozen peaches

- 1 small apple, cored and diced

- 1/2 cucumber, diced

- 1 1/2 cups chopped greens

- 2 tbsp. freshly squeezed lime juice

- 1 1/4 cup coconut water

- handful flat combination of parsley and mint leaves

- A small piece of ginger, peeled

Directions

Combine all the ingredients in a blender and blend on high for about 1 minute or until smooth. Drink it up!

Nutritional information Per Serving:

Calories: 278   Protein: 8.3 g

Total Fat: 3.2 g   Cholesterol: 0 mg

Total Carbs: 26.5 g   Sodium: 96 mg

Dietary Fibre: 15.3 g

Minty Green Smoothie

Yields: 2 Servings

Ingredients

- 1 pear, peeled and chopped

- 3-inch piece cucumber, peeled

- 1/2 lemon, skin on, seeds removed

- 1 cup baby spinach

- 1 stalk kale, stem removed

- A small piece of peeled ginger

- 1 sprig mint leaves

- 1/4 cup fresh parsley

- 1/2 cup water

- Optional: 1 scoop protein powder

Directions

Combine all the ingredients in a blender and blend until very smooth. Enjoy!

Nutritional information Per Serving:

Calories: 122

Protein: 4.9 g

Total Fat: 0.3 g

Cholesterol: 0 mg

Total Carbs: 10.9 g

Sodium: 57 mg

Dietary Fibre: 6.2 g

Grape & Fig Smoothie

Yields: 1 Serving

Ingredients

- 1/3 cup baby spinach

- 1/2 cup red grapes, seeds removed

- 2 figs, the inner flesh scooped out for use

- 1/2 cup purified water

- A pinch of cinnamon

- 5 ice cubes

Directions

Rinse all the ingredients and add to a blender. Blend on high until very smooth. Enjoy!

Nutritional Information Per Serving:

Calories: 204   Dietary fibre: 5.5 g

Total Fat: 0.9 g   Cholesterol: 0 mg

Total Carbs: 52 g   Sodium: 15 mg

Protein: 2.5 g

Citric Berry Smoothie

Yields: 2 Servings

Ingredients

- ¼ tsp. cayenne pepper

- ¼ medium avocado

- 1 tbsp. freshly squeezed lemon juice

- 1 cup chopped fresh kale

- 1 ½ cup coconut water

- 1 cup frozen blueberries

- ½ cup diced mango

- 1 tbsp. ground flaxseed

Directions

Combine everything in a blender and blend until smooth and creamy. Enjoy!

Nutritional Information Per Serving:

Calories: 143

Dietary fibre: 3 g

Total Fat: 1 g

Cholesterol: 0

Total Carbs: 33 g

Sodium: 60 mg

Protein: 4 g

Veggie Cocktail

Yield: 1 Serving

Ingredients

- 3 cups chopped tomatoes

- 2 cups kale

- 2 scallions

- 1 celery rib

- 1/8 tsp. red pepper

- 2 tbsp. freshly squeezed lime juice

- ¼ tsp. minced garlic

- A pinch of sea salt

- ½ cup water

Directions

Blend tomatoes, lime juice, water, and kale in a blend until smooth.

Add garlic, scallions, celery, red pepper and salt and continue blending until very smooth. Serve immediately.

Nutritional Information Per Serving:

Calories: 196

Total Fat: 1.2 g

Total Carbs: 44.9 g

Protein: 9.7 g

Dietary fibre: 9.7 g

Cholesterol: 0

Sodium: 329 mg

Carrot Apple Smoothie

Yield: 1 Serving

Ingredients

- 2 cups baby spinach

- 1 medium apple, cored

- 1 tbsp. freshly grated ginger

- 2 carrots, chopped

- 1 cup filtered water

Directions

Combine all ingredients in a blender until creamy and smooth. Serve right away!

Nutritional Information Per Serving

Calories: 157

Protein: 4 g

Total Fat: 0.6 g

Cholesterol: 0 mg

Total Carbs: 36 g

Sodium: trace

Dietary Fibre: 7 g

Banana Avocado Smoothie

Yield: 1 Serving

Ingredients

- 1-2 cups fresh baby spinach
- 1 celery stick
- 1 apple
- 1 banana
- 1/2 avocado
- 1 cup water

Directions

Combine all the ingredients in a blender and blend until very smooth. Enjoy

Nutritional Information Per Serving

Calories: 365

Protein: 5.2 g

Total Fat: 14 g

Cholesterol: 0 mg

Total Carbs: 61 g

Sodium: 31 mg

Dietary Fibre: 17 g

Pear Wheatgrass Smoothie

Yield: 1 Serving

Ingredients

- 1 pear
- 1/8-ounce wheatgrass
- 2 cups chopped green romaine
- 1/2-inch ginger
- 1 cup water
- 1 cup ice

Directions

Combine all ingredients in a blender and blend until very smooth. Enjoy!

Nutritional Information Per Serving

Calories: 100   Protein: 1.8 g

Total Fat: 0.5 g   Cholesterol: 0 mg

Total Carbs: 24.4 g   Sodium: 10 mg

Dietary Fibre: 6.3 g

Spring Detox Smoothie

Yield: 1 Serving

Ingredients

- 1 cup matcha green tea, chilled

- ½ avocado

- 2 tbsp. freshly squeezed lemon juice

- 1 cup pineapple chunks

- 1 cup cucumber

- 1 cup baby spinach

- 1 tbsp. freshly grated ginger

- 1 cup chopped cilantro

Directions

Combine all ingredients in a blender and blend until very smooth and creamy. Serve right away!

Nutritional Information Per Serving

Calories: 183

Protein: 4 g

Total Fat: 1 g

Cholesterol: 0 mg

Total Carbs: 46 g

Sodium: 31 mg

Dietary Fibre: 5 g

Parting Shot… Maintain the New You!

It's been a long road but you have now learned to eat right and live a healthier life, and there's simply no turning back!

Congratulations for reaching your goal. You have managed to successfully ditch your yo-yo dieting ways and binge eating habits and you are now on a journey of keeping all the good and healthy eating habits that you have learned.

It is now time for us to talk about how to maintain your new and vibrant self before you find yourself spiralling back to where you worked so hard to come from.

To maintain the new, you, we are talking about making permanent lifestyle changes:

Stay positive and realistic

Live life and enjoy every second of it!

Hold on to the satisfaction of being at your dream and healthy weight.

Enjoy little servings of your favourite foods without feeling guilty. And if you do over indulge, cut back a bit and do more exercise the next day as you normally would to balance off the effects. It is all about mindful eating.

Healthy eating is vital! Learn how to choose ingredients, prepare and enjoy a well-balanced meal.

Remember to eat regular meals, take your time to really taste them and indulge yourself occasionally.

Regular physical activity is one of the best things you can do for your body and health.

it will leave you feeling vibrant and energetic to face anything that comes your way. The energizer bunny will be no match for you! Physical activity is an amazing way to beat stress and improve mood so you won't have to crave a tub of ice cream!

After losing weight, the next question is how to maintain your new weight and keep on a healthy track. Here is some piece of advice from an expert:

Never let yourself feel deprived. Switch up your diet and remember to eat in moderation.

Eat out occasionally but remember to be careful with food choices you make. Also, remember to limit fast food.

Continue to eat nutrient dense, balanced and low fat meals with plenty of fruit and veggies.

Sit down in a quiet place to eat your meals. Take time and pay attention to what you eat.

Have three main meals with two or three healthy snacks in between plus 2 glasses of green smoothies to keep your blood sugar levels stable.

Make a conscious decision every day when you wake up to stay on track and keep off all the weight you have lost.

Only eat when you are hungry and find something else to do when you are not hungry to avoid mindless snacking.

Be consistent. Do not set your goals aside on holidays or weekends.

Continue exercising your body on a regular basis. After weight loss, now work on toning your body for a sexy look. Make exercise a natural part of your life and schedule time specifically for it.

Cultivate and maintain healthy relationships with supportive people. Surround yourself with positive energy.

Keep monitoring yourself every now and then to stay conscious of your new healthy habits.

Learn to address your problems without thinking of food.

Enjoy life... you deserve it!

We Are Not a Substitute for a Doctor's Advice

The information contained in this book cannot substitute or replace the services of trained professionals in the field of medical or health matters. In particular, you should consult a physician in all matters relating to mental or physical health, especially concerning symptoms that may require medical attention. This book makes no representation or warranties concerning any treatment of medication. You alone are accountable and responsible for your decisions and consequences in life, and by the use of this book, you agree not to attempt us liable for any such decisions or consequences, at any time, under any circumstances.

Conclusion

Thank you again for reading this book!

I hope this book was able to help you to lose your weight, stay healthy and learn about awesome health benefits.

The next step is to take action.

Again above is a guideline for you to help getting started. Feel free to change the diets according to your desires. If you follow the tips and try the recipes I shared with you, you will definitely see better and a healthier you.

Again thank you for reading this book. Spread the good news and enjoy the Awesome Life style today!

Finally, if you've received value from this book, please take the time to share your thoughts and post a review on Amazon. It'd be greatly appreciated!

Thank you and good luck!

Other Books by Tanya Simons

1) Paleo Diet Cookbook for Beginners

If you are interested in Paleo Diet, this book is the ultimate Guide

This book includes 14 Day Meal Plan to lose 10 lbs in 14 days with 100 Delicious Recipes. Paleo Foods to be taken and Foods to avoid and many more about PALEO Diet Also includes FREE BONUS How to lose weight.

http://www.amazon.com/Paleo-Diet-Beginners-cookbook-Challenge-ebook/dp/B01BT87JVO

2) 10 Day Green Smoothie Cleanse For Weight Loss

Achieve Your Weight Loss Goal and Get Your Figure Back

Lose up to 15 Pounds in 10 Days!

https://www.amazon.com/Day-Green-Smoothie-Cleanse-smoothies-ebook/dp/B01E0LMB6A

3) 10 Day Green Smoothie Cleanse. Delicious Paleo Smoothie Recipes for Weight Loss -Paleo Diet Plan Included.

The basic aim of writing this book is to provide all the weight loss seekers some delicious, scrumptious and mouth-watering green smoothie recipes, which help lose 10 pounds in ten days. If you are a person tired of working out long hours at the gym and feel frustrated following any diet plan, then this 10-day cleanse plan is just for you.

https://www.amazon.com/Day-Green-Smoothie-Cleanse-Delicious-ebook/dp/B01E67VO48

4) Coconut Oil Recipes

Best of Coconut Oil Recipes -Most Delicious Coconut Oil Recipes for Weight loss

http://www.amazon.com/Coconut-Oil-Delicious-Amazingly-Beautiful-ebook/dp/B019KI08KO

5) 60 Most Delicious Coconut Oil Recipes and Amazing Health Benefits for a Perfect Weight Loss.

http://www.amazon.com/Coconut-Oil-Delicious-Benefits-Superfood-ebook/dp/B019E3JHL6

CPSIA information can be obtained
at www.ICGtesting.com
Printed in the USA
LVOW12s0334010617

536512LV00010BA/648/P